YOUR KNOWLEDGE HAS VALUE

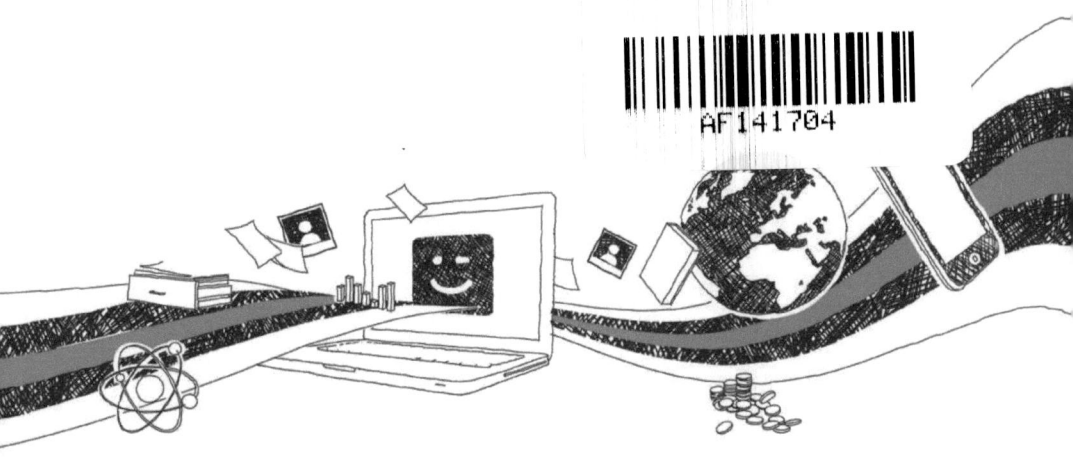
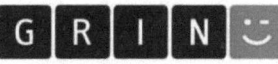

Optimizing Management of PBC-AIH Overlap Syndrome. Insights from the ERN R-LIVER Registry

Anoosha Qaisar

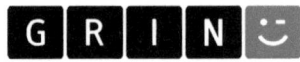

Bibliographic information published by the German National Library:

The German National Library lists this publication in the National Bibliography; detailed bibliographic data are available on the Internet at http://dnb.dnb.de.

ISBN: 9783389102282
This book is also available as an ebook.

© GRIN Publishing GmbH
Trappentreustraße 1
80339 München

Print and binding: Books on Demand GmbH, Norderstedt, Germany
Printed on acid-free paper from responsible sources.

The present work has been carefully prepared. Nevertheless, authors and publishers do not incur liability for the correctness of information, notes, links and advice as well as any printing errors.

GRIN web shop: https://www.grin.com/document/1519338

University of Milano-Bicocca

School of Medicine and Surgery

II Level Master Degree in

Methods and Data AnaLysis (MEDAL) in Biomedical Research

2nd Edition

PBC+AIH syndrome: Survey of the ERN R-LIVER Registry

Candidate: Anoosha Qaisar

Academic year 2022-2023

Acknowledgments

I extend my deepest appreciation to Prof. Maria Grazia Valsecchi and Prof. Stefania Galimberti for graciously welcoming me into their esteemed research group. The opportunity to be a part of this Master program has been truly invaluable, and I am grateful for the knowledge and insights gained during my time with them.

I am indebted to my dedicated supervisors, Dr. Davide Paolo Bernasconi and Dr. Alessio Gerrusi, for their careful guidance and patient intuition throughout the course of my research. Their positive influence and in-depth expertise have significantly shaped my academic journey this year.

My sincere thanks go to Foundazione IRCCS SAN GERARDO DEI TINTORI for providing me with an exceptional opportunity to work alongside top experts in the field of Autoimmune liver diseases. The experience gained in this environment has been instrumental in my growth as a researcher.

I express my gratitude to Prof. Pietro Invernizzi and Dr. Marco Carbone for their valuable contributions to discussions and idea-sharing, enriching my understanding of the subject matter.

A special acknowledgment is reserved for Davide Paolo Bernasconi, whose unwavering support has been a constant source of motivation, particularly during challenging moments. His encouragement has played a pivotal role in my perseverance and success.

I extend heartfelt thanks to my Parents, Siblings and my friend Alessandro Contu for their unwavering support and encouragement, keeping me moving forward at all times.

In conclusion, I am thankful to each individual mentioned for their significant contributions to my academic and personal growth. This journey would not have been as enriching and fulfilling without the support of these exceptional mentors, colleagues, and loved ones.

ABSTRACT

Background & Aims: Primary Biliary Cholangitis (PBC) and Autoimmune Hepatitis (AIH) may show overlapping features in the same individual, challenging clinical management. The aim of this study was to study current disease courses and management of these patients across expert centers in Europe.

Methods: Data from the prospective R-LIVER registry of the European Reference Network (ERN)-RARE LIVER were analyzed. The dataset included newly diagnosed patients with AIH treated with Ursodeoxycholic Acid (UDCA) (group A), PBC receiving immunosuppression (IS) (group B), PBC on UDCA (group C), PBC and AIH (group D), from 2017 to 2023. Clinical features and treatment regimens at diagnosis and after 12 and 24 months were compared across groups. Transitions in treatment regimens over time were depicted by alluvial plots. A decision tree (DT) algorithm was used to reclassify patients into groups based on clinical features at diagnosis.

Results:
In this study, 372 individuals with a median follow-up of 24 months were analyzed across the four groups. Group A included 23 cases, group B 8 cases, group C 306 cases and group D included 35 cases. At diagnosis, patients in group D showed higher median AST, ALT, IgG, IgM values than patients in group B and C. At follow-up and after treatment, differences in AST, ALT, IgG and IgM values disappeared; yet, patients in group B showed persistently higher elevated levels of ALP and GGT as compared to group D. Treatment regimens changed for all groups, with 77% of PBC and AIH cases remaining on UDCA + IS during the 2nd follow-up, while 56% in Group A remained stable on the same treatment. Decision tree-based classification showed a high agreement with the clinical diagnosis groups (accuracy 87.7% on the test set).

Conclusion: Patients with PBC and AIH have different biochemical features at diagnosis as compared to patients with single disease phenotypes. Yet, the lack of well-defined clinical pathways generates significant heterogeneity in treatment regimens. Further agreement among experts and prospective studies are needed to optimize management strategies for this complex patient population.

Key Words: autoimmunity, liver, overlap syndromes, immunosuppression, precision medicine.

Table of contents

Chapter 1: Introduction and Aims of study

1.1 Definition and epidemiology of PBC-AIH syndrome

Autoimmune Hepatitis (AIH) and Primary Biliary Cholangitis (PBC) stand as distinct immune-mediated liver diseases, each characterized by a unique set of clinical, biochemical, serological, and histological parameters. However, the intricate landscape of autoimmune liver disorders occasionally blurs the lines between these conditions, giving rise to overlap syndromes.

These enigmatic overlap syndromes manifest when auto-antibodies, clinical presentations, and serological findings coalesce in combinations that defy the conventional boundaries of AIH and PBC. Recognizing and understanding these elusive overlap syndromes is of paramount clinical significance, since it profoundly influences treatment strategies.

PBC-AIH overlap syndrome predominantly affects women, with 83 to 100% of reported cases being female. The average age at diagnosis is around 45 years, ranging from 38 to 56 years. This syndrome is observed across various ethnicities. Diagnosis can be challenging due to nonspecific clinical manifestations that overlap with other liver diseases.[2]

1.2 Diagnosis

The Paris criteria, developed by Chazouillères et al, are commonly used for diagnosing PBC-AIH overlap syndrome (Figure 1). These criteria require the presence of at least two out of three diagnostic criteria for both PBC and AIH. For PBC, the criteria include elevated alkaline phosphatases and/or GGT levels, the presence of anti-mitochondrial antibodies, and histological evidence of destructive lymphocytic cholangitis. For AIH, criteria involve elevated ALT levels, increased IgG levels, the presence of anti-smooth muscle antibodies, and liver histology showing marked periportal and lobular inflammatory lesions.[3,4]

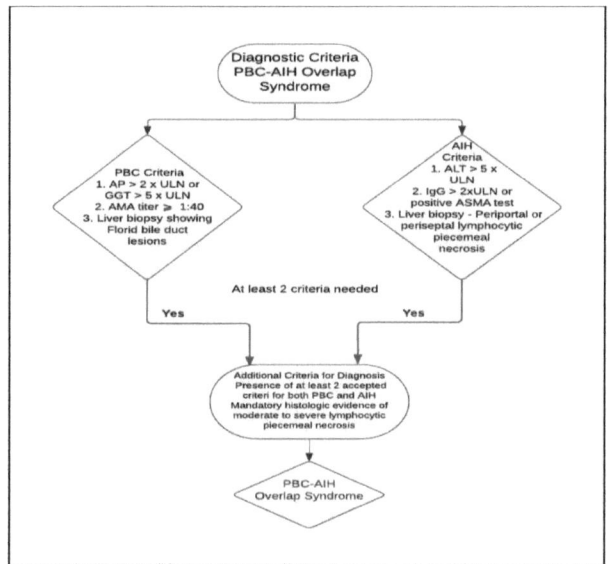

Figure 1: Diagnostic PARIS criteria of PBC+AIH overlap syndrome.

While these criteria lack a gold standard for validation, they are widely accepted, and are practical for implementation due to their simplicity and precision. The European Association for the Study of Liver (EASL) endorses these criteria.[5]

Retrospective assessments indicate the presence of this specific variant in 5% of Autoimmune Hepatitis (AIH) cases and 19% of Primary Biliary Cholangitis (PBC) cases. The diagnostic framework described lacks a well-defined sensitivity for identifying the syndrome, yet it presents a consistent and broadly applicable diagnostic model. An alternative strategy suggests categorizing individuals with cumulative scores surpassing 10, positive anti-mitochondrial antibody (AMA) seropositivity, and histological signs of cholangitis as PBC+AIH variants.[6]

In the realm of primary biliary cholangitis (PBC), the detection of antinuclear antibodies in serum does not mean PBC-AIH overlap. Recently, a scoring system for PBC has been proposed with the aim of distinguishing PBC from overlapping and outlier autoimmune hepatic cholangiopathies. Despite its appeal, the utility of this model necessitates validation through cross-evaluation before its implementation in clinical settings.[7]

It has been observed that genetically predisposed AIH patients may experience an exacerbation of autoimmune bile duct damage, resulting in a mixed clinical presentation of both AIH and PBC features. This complex interplay may significantly impact the course of the disease, although the clinical significance of this categorization remains uncertain.[8]

1.3 Prognosis

Research findings on patients with overlap syndromes reveal diverse outcomes. Some studies point to a swift advancement towards cirrhosis and liver failure, while others highlight an increased chance of developing esophageal varices, ascites, and liver failure compared to those with typical PBC. Both scenarios indicate higher risks of disease progression.

1.4 Treatment

The diagnosis of an overlap syndrome has therapeutic implications. Traditional immunosuppression is a standard treatment for AIH, while UDCA is recommended to slow the progression of PBC. A combination therapy of UDCA and corticosteroids has shown success in achieving a complete clinical and biochemical response in patients with overlap PBC+AIH.[8,9]

In a German study, a group of patients, numbering 20 each for AIH, PBC, and PBC+AIH overlap, exhibited clinical features consistent with primary biliary cholangitis (PBC), including the presence of AMA-M2 antibodies and characteristic bile duct damage. However, they also displayed a more hepatitis-like presentation and showed a favorable response to corticosteroid treatment.[13]

Both EASL and the American Association for the Study of Liver Diseases (AASLD) recommend the use of combination therapy with corticosteroids and UDCA for PBC+AIH overlap syndrome. However, it is essential to note that this recommendation is not strongly evidence-based, and the effectiveness of this treatment varies widely, likely due to differences in diagnostic criteria and dosing schedules. Corticosteroids alone have produced inconsistent results, mycophenolate mofetil has shown little efficacy, and calcineurin inhibitors have rarely been used in this context.[10,11,12]

1.5 Aims of the study

Our study delves into the clinical presentation and therapeutic outcomes of adult patients diagnosed with the PBC+AIH variant syndrome over a two-year follow-up period. Utilizing data from the European Reference Network (ERN) registry, we aimed to provide insights into the diagnostic practices, biochemical response rates, and comparative features among patients with PBC+AIH overlap as compared to other variants of PBC and AIH.

This research project addresses two key aims: comparing features of PBC+AIH patients with other diagnostic groups and evaluating biochemical response rates at 12 and 24 months

Chapter 2: Patients and methods

2.1 Description of the dataset

In this study, the prospective R-LIVER registry of the European Reference Network (ERN)-RARE LIVER was analyzed. The dataset includes newly diagnosed patients with AIH treated with Ursodeoxycholic Acid (UDCA) (group A), PBC receiving immunosuppression (IS) (group B), PBC on UDCA (group C), PBC and AIH (group D), since 2017 to 2023. The extensive dataset comprised clinical, laboratory, and histological information collected at the time of initial diagnosis and subsequent follow-up intervals, spanning 12 months, and 24 months. Retrospective data up to 12 months from the time of diagnosis were considered, with ongoing annual follow-ups recorded within the registry. The documentation of PBC+AIH overlap syndrome and associated clinical complications adhered to international definitions established at the inception of the registry

To ensure a robust cohort, inclusion criteria were applied, and records with less than 12 months of follow-up were excluded. This culling process refined the study population to include data from ten remaining centers. Data handling practices included no imputation for missing values, and statistical analyses were adjusted for center-specific reference values. The study maintained adherence to the diagnostic and severity criteria recently published by ERN registry.[15] This comprehensive and refined approach aims to contribute a nuanced understanding of the clinical and biochemical characteristics of PBC+AIH overlap syndrome in comparison to other pertinent groups in the study.

2.2 Data analysis

The analyses were carried out using R software version 4.3.2. Box-plots were used to show the distribution of biochemical variables including AST,ALT,IgG,GGT,ALP,IgM and IgA.

The Wilcoxon-Mann-Whitney test with Bonferroni adjustment was used to compare the distribution of the variables between groups pairwise. To provide a graphical representation of the treatments administered to patients of the four groups at the three time points, an alluvial plot was generated.[16]

2.3 Selection of variables and imputation of missing data

For the aim of this analysis patients have been categorized into three groups: those receiving AIH treatment with UDCA (56 patients), those solely diagnosed with PBC (671 patients), and those diagnosed with both PBC and AIH (62 patients).

The selection of variables for analysis was driven by clinical relevance, focusing on parameters commonly associated with liver function and autoimmune liver diseases. Variables such as liver enzymes (AST, ALT), bilirubin levels, biomarkers (γ-GT, IGG, IGA, IGM), and antibody tests (Anti-AMA, Anti-ANA) were chosen due to their diagnostic significance in liver disorders. Missing data were imputed using the Multiple Imputation by Chained Equations (MICE) algorithm using the eponymous R package.[17]

This package employs multiple imputation by chained equations (MICE) to estimate missing values based on observed data, preserving the underlying structure and relationships within the dataset. By using MICE imputation, the integrity of the dataset was maintained, enabling more robust analysis and interpretation of results in the context of autoimmune liver diseases.

2.4 Machine learning supervised classification of diagnosis groups
Following the imputation process, the dataset was randomly split into distinct training (70% of the observations) and test (30% of the observations) sets. After splitting the dataset into training and testing sets, the model was trained using the caret package and the rpart method. Supervised machine learning involves the training of a model on labeled data, where the algorithm learns to make predictions based on input variables and known outcomes.

2.5 Decision tree Classification model
A decision tree classification was performed to distinguish between different groups of patients based on clinical and demographic variables., which is a popular supervised learning technique used to classify data into categories or predict outcomes.[18] In decision tree classification, the algorithm learns from the data by recursively splitting the dataset into subsets based on the values of input features. At each step, the algorithm selects the feature that best separates the data into distinct categories, optimizing for maximum information gain or purity of the subsets. This process continues until the data is effectively partitioned into homogeneous groups, or until a stopping criterion is met.

Once the decision tree is constructed, it can be used to classify new data by traversing the tree from the root node down to a leaf node, where a decision or prediction is made based on the majority class of the instances in that node. Decision trees are particularly intuitive and interpretable, as they mimic the human decision-making process by following a series of logical steps to reach a conclusion.

In the context of this study, decision tree classification was employed to predict the diagnosis groups based on the clinical and biochemical baseline characteristics of patients. The decision tree was built on the training dataset and the performance was evaluated on the test set.

This strategic approach not only enhances the reliability of the analysis but also contributes significantly to the understanding of the clinical and biochemical characteristics of PBC+AIH overlap syndrome. By leveraging machine learning techniques, we can glean deeper insights into the nuances of this complex medical condition, thereby paving the way for more informed decision-making and tailored patient care strategies.

Chapter 3: Results

3.1 Study population

Data were collected prospectively from the launch of the R-LIVER registry in 2017 until 2023. The dataset includes 968 adult patients. Among them, 372 patients with at least 12 months of follow-up were included in our investigation and classified in distinct groups according to diagnosis and treatment received: "AIH ON UDCA" (n=23), "PBC ON IS" (n=8), "PBC ON UDCA" (n=306), and "PBC+AIH" (n=35) . Analysis revealed significant variations in demographic parameters.

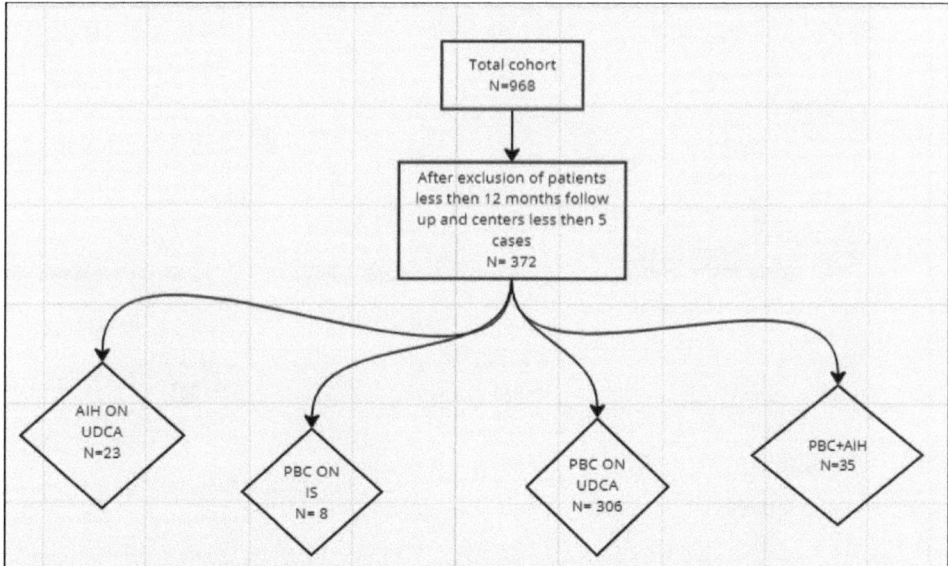

Figure 2.This flowchart highlights gender heterogeneity among our study cohorts.

Patients diagnosed with AIH while on UDCA had a mean age of 47.91(20.49) years, while those with PBC on immunosuppression had the highest mean age at 59.12 (12.48) years. PBC patients on UDCA and those with PBC+AIH had mean ages of 55.72(11.22) and 52.80(12.67) years, respectively (p-value = 0.013). Sex distribution varied across groups, with AIH ON UDCA predominantly female (82.6%) and PBC ON IS predominantly female (87.5%). PBC ON UDCA and PBC+AIH groups had even higher female percentages (91.2% and 74.3%, respectively), with a significant difference among groups (p-value = 0.017). These findings highlight age and gender heterogeneity among our study cohorts.

3.2 Biochemical responses

In examining the biochemical markers across different groups of patients with autoimmune liver diseases, distinct patterns emerge, particularly notable when comparing the group with the coexistence of Primary Biliary Cholangitis (PBC) and Autoimmune Hepatitis (AIH) (PBC+AIH) with the other three groups. As shown in figure 3 below Aspartate Aminotransferase (AST) levels at diagnosis , Patients with AIH on Ursodeoxycholic Acid (UDCA) exhibit a significantly higher median level (490.00 [IQR: 72.50, 611.00]) compared to those with PBC+AIH (101.00 [51.00, 246.50]), PBC on UDCA (43.00 [27.00, 65.00]), and PBC on immunosuppression (IS) (120.00 [84.75, 391.75]) (p < 0.001). A similar trend is observed during follow-up at both 12 and 24 months, suggesting sustained differences in AST levels. Alanine Aminotransferase (ALT) levels at diagnosis also follow a similar trend, with AIH ON UDCA patients having higher levels compared to the other groups (p < 0.001). This pattern persists during follow-up at 12 months but becomes less pronounced at 24 months.

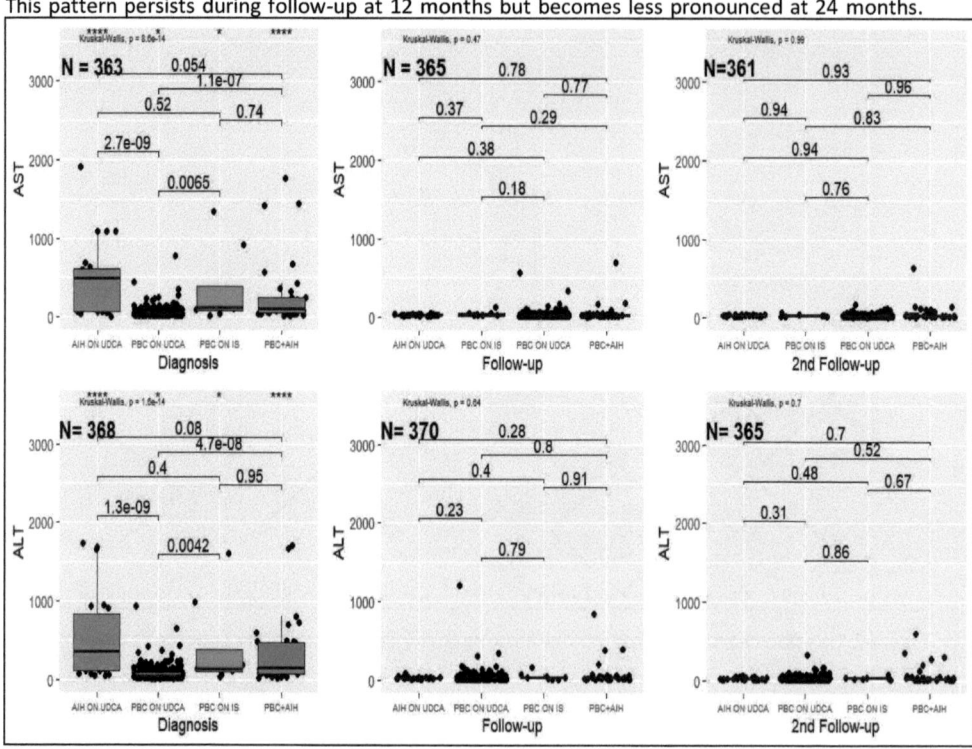

Figure 3: Box-plots of Aspartate Aminotransferase(AST) and Alanine Aminotransferase(ALT) by group at the three time points.

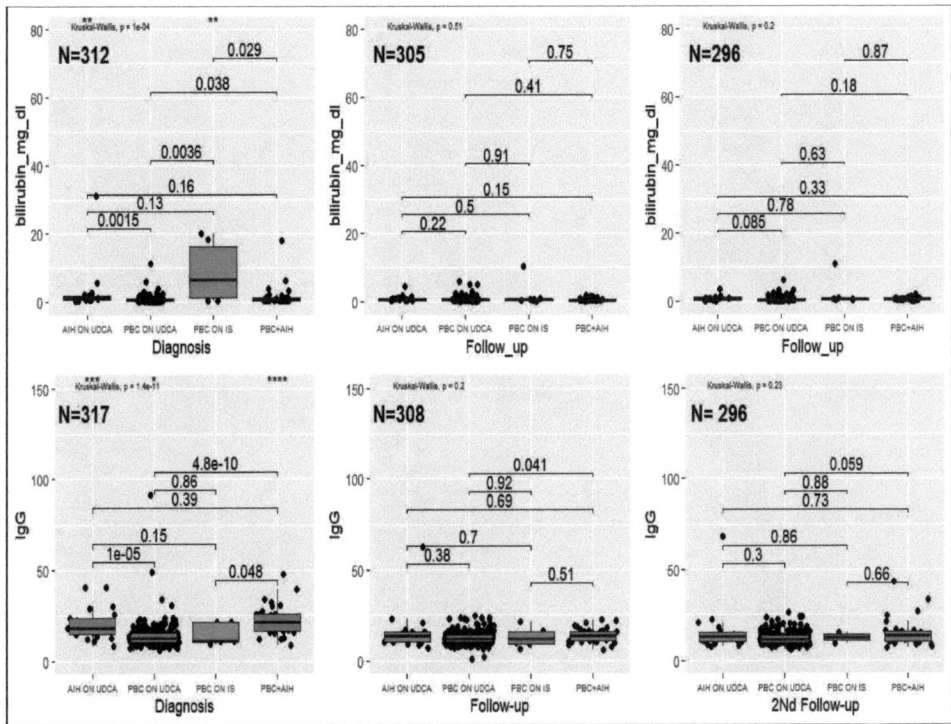

Figure 4: Box-plots of Immunoglobulin G(igG) and bilirubin mg/dl by group at the three time points.

As shown in figure 4. Immunoglobulin G (IgG) levels at diagnosis are significantly higher in PBC+AIH patients compared to the other groups (p < 0.001). The bilirubin levels at diagnosis for PBC+AIH patients are 0.70 [IQR: 0.49, 1.30], not significantly different from other groups (p = 0.204), indicating comparable levels of liver dysfunction.

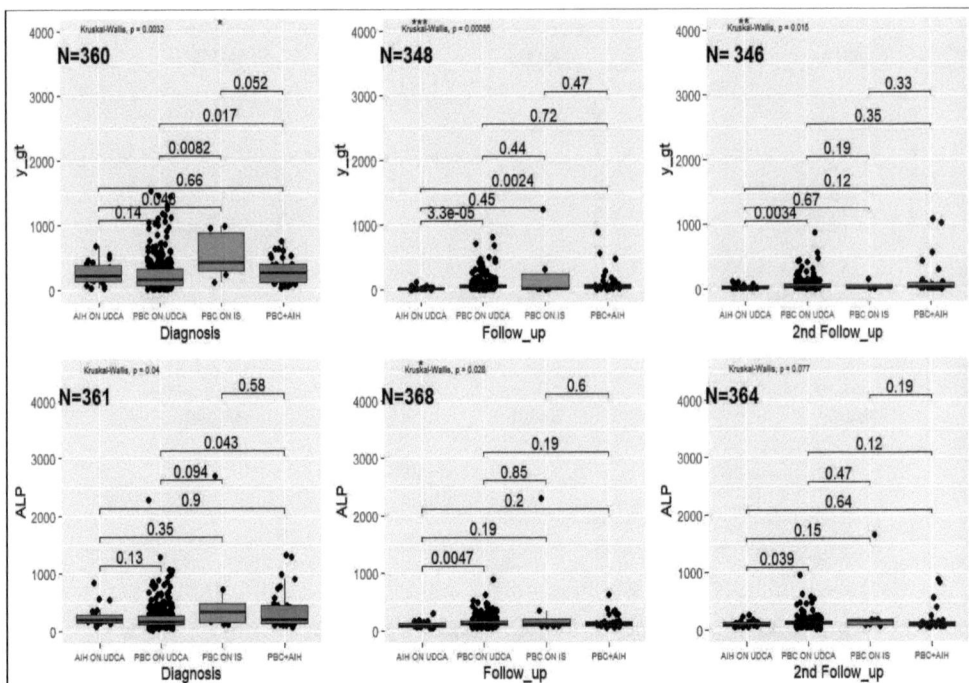

Figure 5 : Box-plots of Alkaline phosphatase(ALP) and gamma-glutamyl transferase(yGT) by group at the three time points.

Furthermore, In figure 5 Alkaline phosphatase(ALP) levels at diagnosis are also significantly different among the groups (p = 0.04), with PBC+AIH patients showing higher levels compared to those with AIH on UDCA and PBC on UDCA. Similarly, gamma-glutamyl transferase (yGT) levels at diagnosis are significantly higher in the PBC+AIH group and PBC ON IS group compared to the other groups (p = 0.003), indicating greater liver cell damage or cholestasis.

Overall, these findings underscore distinct biochemical profiles in patients with PBC+AIH compared to those with singular autoimmune liver diseases, emphasizing the complexity and potential severity of the overlapping syndrome. Specifically, in addition to elevated IgG levels, significant differences are observed in ALP and GGT levels, indicative of varied immunological and hepatic responses.

When considering disease progression, the levels of AST, ALT, ALP, and bilirubin tend to decrease over follow-up periods in all groups, indicating a positive response to treatment. However, there are subtle differences in the rate of improvement among the groups. Patients with PBC+AIH often demonstrate a trajectory of biochemical improvement that falls between that of PBC and AIH alone, further highlighting the complex interplay of these conditions in disease progression.

Moreover, the degree of hepatocellular injury, as indicated by the levels of AST, ALT, and IgG, appears to be more pronounced in patients with the overlap syndrome, suggesting a synergistic effect of both diseases on liver function.

3.3 Treatment protocols

The breakdown of treatments among four distinct groups: AIH ON UDCA, PBC ON UDCA, PBC ON immunosuppression(IS), and PBC+AIH reveals a nuanced landscape of medication regimens and follow-up trends. In the AIH ON UDCA group, 20 patients received both treatments, while 3 opted for PBC treatment alone. At 12 and 24 months follow-up, the variability in treatment persists, with 15 patients continuing with both treatments, 5 receiving immunosuppression only at 12 months, and 12 remaining on dual therapy at 24 months. Conversely, PBC ON UDCA predominantly relies on PBC treatment alone, with 283 patients receiving this sole treatment, and only 23 patients receiving no treatment as shown in figure 6.

In contrast, both PBC ON immunosuppression(PBC ON IS) and PBC+AIH show intermittent utilization of dual therapy, with 7 patients in PBC ON IS and 25 patients in PBC+AIH receiving both treatments initially. However, at subsequent follow-ups, the number of patients on dual therapy fluctuates. These findings underscore the complexity of managing autoimmune liver diseases and emphasize the importance of personalized strategies in optimizing patient outcomes.

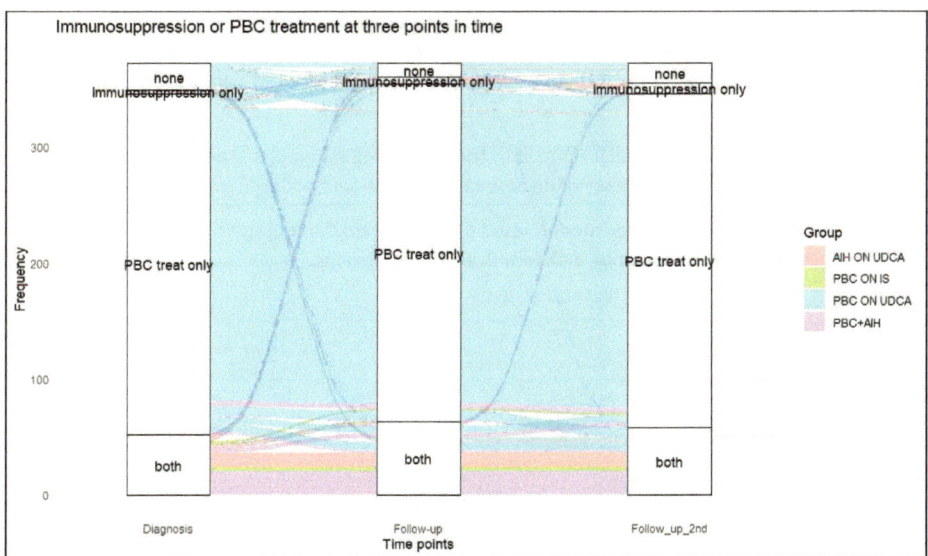

Figure 6: Alluvial Plot
The alluvial plot shows how different treatments were given to 372 patients with various diagnoses at different time points. It helps us see which diagnoses were more common and which treatments were used most often. It also shows how patients' treatments changed over time, like if they switched to different treatments at follow-up appointments. Basically, the alluvial plot gives us a simple and clear picture of how diagnoses, treatments, and patient outcomes are connected in our study group.

The resulting Decision tree Classification model achieved an overall accuracy of approximately 87.7% on the test set, indicating a relatively good predictive performance.Specifically, the model was able to accurately classify patients into their respective liver disease categories, such as primary biliary cholangitis (PBC), autoimmune hepatitis (AIH) ON UDCA, and PBC+AIH overlap syndrome This level of accuracy was observed when evaluating the model's performance on a separate test dataset.

Upon examining the confusion matrix, it's evident that the model performed reasonably well in predicting patients with PBC, achieving a sensitivity of 95.5%, and those with AIH, achieving a sensitivity of 62.5%. However, the sensitivity for predicting patients with the combined condition of PBC+AIH was lower at 22.2%.The fact that patients of this group are the most difficult to be identified seems logical, because PBC+AIH is the overlapping syndrome and thus it is hard to distinguish them from PBC and from AIH. The specificity was high across all classes, indicating a low rate of false positives.

The most important variables identified by the model for classification included laboratory parameters such as alanine aminotransferase(ALT) and aspartate aminotransferase(AST) levels, indicating their significant contribution to distinguishing between different liver disease groups. Additionally, variables related to diagnostic procedures, such as liver biopsy at diagnosis and the requirement for specific antibody tests (e.g., anti-AMA), also contributed significantly to the classification process.

These procedures provided crucial insights into the underlying pathological and immunological mechanisms, enhancing the accuracy of disease classification and patient stratification.

In summary, the classification tree model based on clinical and demographic variables showed promising performance in predicting different liver disease groups.

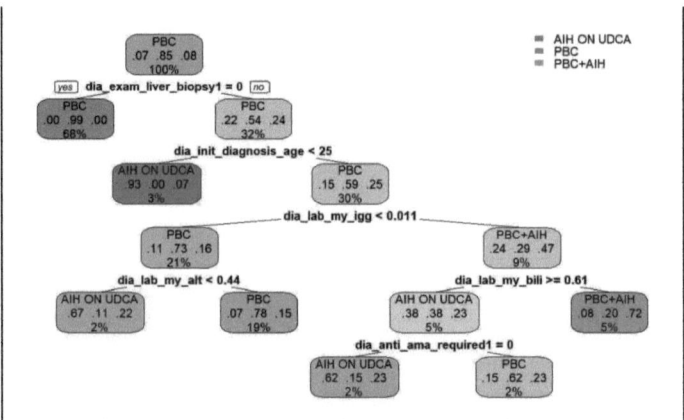

Figure 7: Graphical representation of the decision tree applied to the test set.

The decision tree analysis begins with assigning patients to the most prevalent category which is PBC group. If a patient thus does not undergo liver biopsy, it will be assigned again to the PBC category while the remaining patients will proceed to the following leaves.

Patients younger than 25 years are assigned to the AIH in the UDCA category. The other patients will be split based on the IGG value. If the value (X ULN) is lower than 0.011, then ALT should be checked and if this is lower than 0.44 X ULN the patient is assigned to AIH on UDCA, otherwise the patient is assigned to the PBC category. Patients with IgG>0.011 are then assigned to the PBC+AIH category if the bilirubin is lower than 0.61 X ULN. Those with higher bilirubin are split based on a test of ama antibodies: if the test was negative they are assigned to AIH on UDCA, otherwise to PBC.

Chapter 4: Discussion and conclusions

Based on the comprehensive analysis conducted in this study, several key findings and conclusions can be drawn regarding the management and prognosis of patients with PBCand AIH.

Firstly, the examination of biochemical tests, including liver enzymes such as ALT, ALP, and bilirubin, revealed important associations with disease progression and treatment response. For example, elevated ALT levels were found to be associated with certain treatment modalities, such as UDCA and immunosuppression, suggesting their potential efficacy in managing liver inflammation and disease activity.

Secondly, the decision tree algorithm effectively predicted patient subgroups based on specific clinical and biochemical parameters. It successfully stratified individuals into distinct categories corresponding to primary biliary cholangitis (PBC), autoimmune hepatitis (AIH) on UDCA, and PBC+AIH overlap syndrome. This predictive capability offers valuable insights for clinicians in tailoring treatment strategies to individual patient profiles, potentially leading to more effective management and improved outcomes for those with complex liver disorders.
However, further refinement and validation of the model may be necessary to improve its sensitivity, particularly for identifying patients with complex conditions such as PBC+AIH.

This study highlights the complexity of PBC and AIH management and underscores the need for personalized treatment approaches tailored to individual patient profiles. By integrating decision tree analysis, biochemical tests, treatment strategies, and regression modeling, this research contributes to a better understanding of disease mechanisms and provides valuable insights into optimizing patient care.

For future research, expanding the dataset to include a larger and more diverse patient population could further enhance the generalizability of the findings. Additionally, incorporating novel biomarkers and advanced imaging techniques may offer additional insights into disease progression and treatment response. Furthermore, longitudinal studies tracking patients over time could provide valuable information on the long-term efficacy and safety of different treatment modalities. Overall, continued research in this field is essential for improving the management and outcomes of patients with PBC and AIH. Additionally, leveraging artificial intelligence techniques can further optimize disease prediction, treatment selection, and patient monitoring in PBC and AIH management.

References:

1.Bairy, Indira. "Autoimmune Hepatitis – Primary Biliary Cirrhosis Overlap Syndrome." JOURNAL OF CLINICAL AND DIAGNOSTIC RESEARCH, 2017. DOI.org (Crossref), https://doi.org/10.7860/JCDR/2017/25193.10242.

2.Razafindrazoto,Chantelli lamblaudiot, et al. "Primary Biliary Cholangitis-autoimmune Hepatitis Overlap Syndrome: Case Report and Literature Review." Clinical Case Reports, vol. 9, no. 3, Mar. 2021, pp. 1647–50. DOI.org (Crossref), https://doi.org/10.1002/ccr3.3861.

3.Chazouillères, Olivier, et al. "Primary Biliary Cirrhosis-Autoimmune Hepatitis Overlap Syndrome: Clinical Features and Response to Therapy: Primary Biliary Cirrhosis-Autoimmune Hepatitis Overlap Syndrome: Clinical Features and Response to Therapy." Hepatology, vol. 28, no. 2, Aug. 1998, pp. 296–301. DOI.org (Crossref), https://doi.org/10.1002/hep.510280203.

4.Talwalkar, Jayant A., et al. "Overlap of Autoimmune Hepatitis and Primary Biliary Cirrhosis: An Evaluation of a Modified Scoring System." The American Journal of Gastroenterology, vol. 97, no. 5, May 2002, pp. 1191–97. DOI.org (Crossref), https://doi.org/10.1111/j.1572-0241.2002.05703.x.

5.European Association for the Study of the Liver. "EASL Clinical Practice Guidelines: Management of Cholestatic Liver Diseases." Journal of Hepatology, vol. 51, no. 2, Aug. 2009, pp. 237–67. DOI.org (Crossref), https://doi.org/10.1016/j.jhep.2009.04.009.

6.Ben-Ari, Z. "Autoimmune Hepatitis and Its Variant Syndromes." Gut, vol. 49, no. 4, Oct. 2001, pp. 589–94. DOI.org (Crossref), https://doi.org/10.1136/gut.49.4.589.

7.Beuers, Ulrich. "Hepatic Overlap Syndromes." Journal of Hepatology, vol. 42, no. 1, Apr. 2005, pp. S93–99. DOI.org (Crossref), https://doi.org/10.1016/j.jhep.2004.11.009.

8.Boberg, Kirsten Muri, et al. "Overlap Syndromes: The International Autoimmune Hepatitis Group (IAIHG) Position Statement on a Controversial Issue." Journal of Hepatology, vol. 54, no. 2, Feb. 2011, pp. 374–85. DOI.org (Crossref), https://doi.org/10.1016/j.jhep.2010.09.002.

9.Czaja, Albert J. "The Overlap Syndromes of Autoimmune Hepatitis." Digestive Diseases and Sciences, Aug. 2012. DOI.org (Crossref), https://doi.org/10.1007/s10620-012-2367-1

10.Czaja, Albert J. "Diagnosis and Management of the Overlap Syndromes of Autoimmune Hepatitis." Canadian Journal of Gastroenterology, vol. 27, no. 7, 2013, pp. 417–23. DOI.org (Crossref), https://doi.org/10.1155/2013/198070.

11.Czaja, Albert J. "Frequency and Nature of the Variant Syndromes of Autoimmune Liver Disease." Hepatology, vol. 28, no. 2, Aug. 1998, pp. 360–65. DOI.org (Crossref), https://doi.org/10.1002/hep.510280210.

12.Lohse AW, zum Büschenfelde KH, Franz B, Kanzler S, Gerken G, Dienes HP. Characterization of the overlap syndrome of primary biliary cirrhosis (PBC) and autoimmune hepatitis: evidence for it being a hepatitic form of PBC in genetically susceptible individuals. Hepatology. 1999;29:1078-1084.

13.Freedman, Benjamin L., et al. "Treatment of Overlap Syndromes in Autoimmune Liver Disease: A Systematic Review and Meta-Analysis." Journal of Clinical Medicine, vol. 9, no. 5, May 2020, p. 1449. DOI.org (Crossref), https://doi.org/10.3390/jcm9051449.

14.Czaja, Albert J. "The Variant Forms of Autoimmune Hepatitis." Annals of Internal Medicine, vol. 125, no. 7, Oct. 1996, p. 588. DOI.org (Crossref), https://doi.org/10.7326/0003-4819-125-7-199610010-00009.

15."Registry."Rare-Liver.Eu,https://rare-liver.eu/healthcare-professionals/registry/.

16.Jason Cory Brunson and Quentin D. Read (2023). ggalluvial: Alluvial Plots in 'ggplot2'. R package version 0.12.5. Alluvial Plots in Ggplot2. https://corybrunson.github.io/ggalluvial/.

17.Buuren, Stef Van, and Karin Groothuis-Oudshoorn. "Mice : Multivariate Imputation by Chained Equations in R." Journal of Statistical Software, vol. 45, no. 3, 2011. DOI.org (Crossref), https://doi.org/10.18637/jss.v045.i03.

18.James, Gareth, et al. An Introduction to Statistical Learning: With Applications in R. 2013.

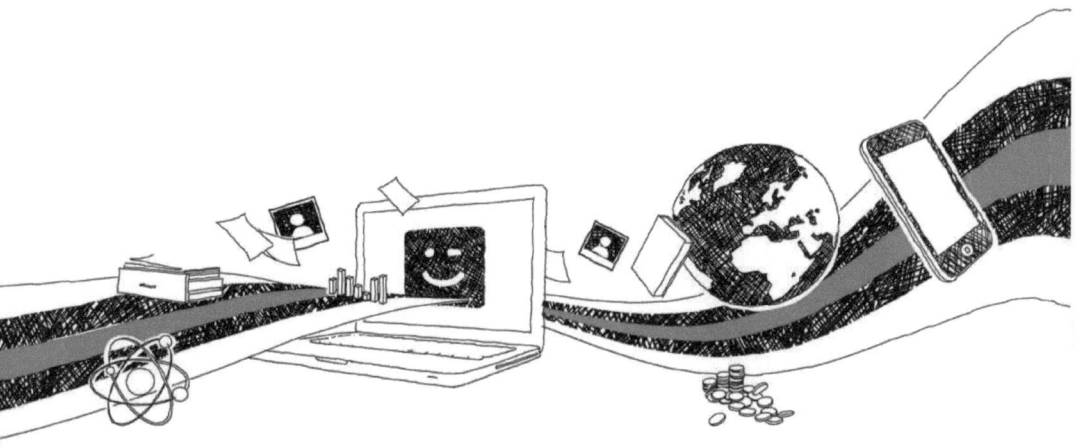
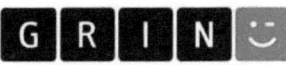